The Must-Have Pregnancy Cookbook

The Guide to a Healthy Pregnancy

BY: Allie Allen

COOK & ENJOY

Copyright 2019 Allie Allen

Copyright Notes

This book is written as an informational tool. While the author has taken every precaution to ensure the accuracy of the information provided therein, the reader is warned that they assume all risk when following the content. The author will not be held responsible for any damages that may occur as a result of the readers' actions.

The author does not give permission to reproduce this book in any form, including but not limited to: print, social media posts, electronic copies or photocopies, unless permission is expressly given in writing.

Table of Contents

Delicious Recipes for Optimum Pregnancy

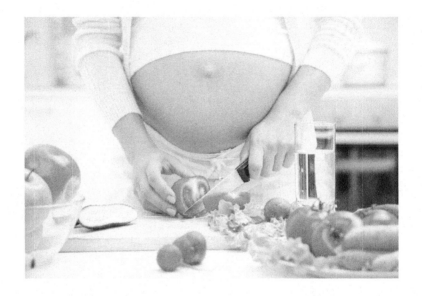

sssssssssssssssssssssssssssssssssssssssssssssssssssss

1) Energized Meatloaf

Who says that you can't enjoy meatloaf, even if it is done bulletproof style? This meatloaf recipe will surely impress all of your guests and will leave them wanting more.

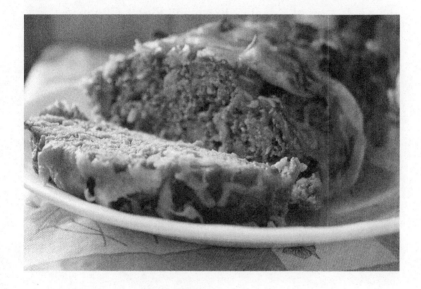

Cooking Time: 55 Minutes

Makes: 6 to 8

List of Ingredients:

- 2 Eggs, Large in Size and Pastured
- 1 Pound of Beef, Grass Fed
- 1 Onion, Medium in Size, Red and Chopped Finely
- 2 Cloves of Garlic, Minced
- ¼ Cup of Cilantro, Fresh and Finely Chopped
- ½ Cup of Parsley, Fresh and Finely Chopped
- ½ Of a Red Pepper, Peeled, Deseeded and Finely Chopped
- Dash of Sea Salt and Pepper for Taste
- 1 teaspoon of Cumin, Powder
- 1 tablespoon of Coconut Oil

ssssssssssssssssssssssssssssssssssssssssssssssssss

Procedure:

1. Leave your oven to preheat at 350 degrees. While it heats up take out a baking dish and line it with some baking paper (parchment paper) and set aside.

2. Next take out a large sized bowl and add all of your ingredients, including the pastured eggs, onion, ground beef, the herbs and garlic and cumin powder. Season with your dash of salt and pepper and mix together until combined well.

3. Once everything is evenly combined, take out the baking tray you prepared earlier and place your mixture into it.

4. Then pop it into your oven and cook for the 45 minutes or until the meatloaf starts turning golden brown in color.

5. Then use a skewer to pierce and test the center of the meatloaf. If it isn't fully cooked, bake for an additional 10 minutes.

6. Serve with a light salad or bowl of steamed vegetables and enjoy thoroughly.

2) Filling Garlic and Cauliflower Soup

While cauliflower is relatively mild in flavor, it can take a lot of seasoning in order to make it taste better. No better seasoning helps than garlic and some black pepper. This soup is an extremely creamy and savory soup, which will surely please even the pickiest of eaters.

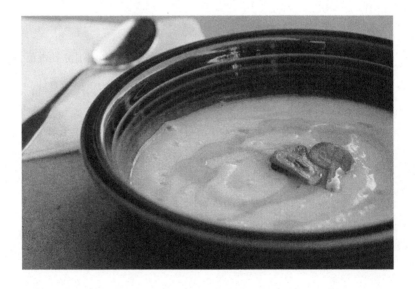

Cooking Time: 45 Minutes

Makes: 6 Servings

List of Ingredients:

- 2 Tablespoons of Olive Oil
- 1 Onion, Medium in Size and Finely Chopped
- 4 Cloves of Garlic, Finely Chopped
- 1 Head of Cauliflower, Fresh and Sliced into Florets
- 4 Cups of Vegetable Stock, Low in Sodium
- Dash of Salt and Pepper for Taste
- ½ of a Lemon, Fresh and Juiced
- ¼ teaspoons of Cumin Powder, Ground

ssssssssssssssssssssssssssssssssssssssssssssssssssss

Procedure:

1. Using a large sized soup pot, heat up your olive oil and add in your minced garlic and chopped onion. Sauté them both for the next 2 minutes or until fragrant.

2. Next add in your cauliflower and vegetable stock. Season with your dash of salt and pepper. On medium heat allow your soup to cook for the next 20 minutes.

3. After 20 minutes add in your cumin powder and fresh lemon juice. Remove from heat and transfer soup into a blender. Puree your soup until it reaches the desired consistency.

4. Pour into a few serving bowls and serve while still warm. Enjoy.

3) Fresh Bakes Green Chilies and Tomatoes with Quinoa

If you are a fan of stuffed tomatoes, then you are going to love this dish. This recipe includes stuffed tomatoes that are packed full of healthy quinoa and sweet corn. It is covered with melted cheese which will surely leave your guests mouths watering.

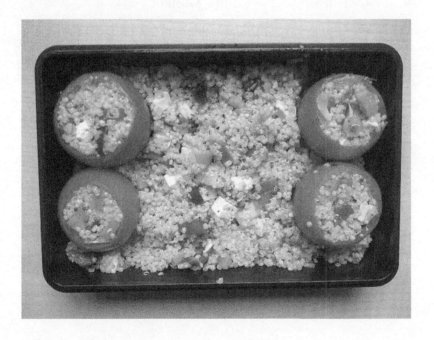

Cooking Time: 1 Hour and 5 Minutes

Makes: 6

List of Ingredients:

- 2 Poblano Chilies, Finely Chopped
- 2 Cups of Corn Kernels, Fresh
- 1 Cup of Onion, Chopped Finely
- 1 tablespoon of Oregano, Fresh and Chopped Finely
- 1 tablespoon of Olive Oil
- 1 tablespoon of Lime Juice, Fresh
- 1 teaspoon of Salt, Evenly Divided
- ¾ teaspoons of Cumin, Ground
- ¼ teaspoons of Black Pepper, Ground and Fresh
- 6 Tomatoes, Ripe
- 1 Cup of Quinoa, Uncooked
- ¼ Cup of Water
- 4 Ounces of Colby Jack Cheese, Shredded

sssssssssssssssssssssssssssssssssssssssssssssssss

Procedure:

1. Preheat your oven to broiler. While this heats up prepare your chilies by slicing them in half lengthwise and clean out the insides. Place your chilies onto a baking sheet and broil for at least 8 minutes or until the chilies are fully blackened. Remove from heat and chop your chilies finely.

2. Add in your onions and corn to your baking pan and place into your oven to broil to cook for 10 minutes, making sure to stir at least twice. Once done add to your chopped-up chilies. Add in your lime juice, black pepper, oregano, salt and cumin and toss lightly to combine thoroughly. Set aside.

3. Next cut the tops of your tomatoes and set the tops aside. Being as careful as you can scoop out your tomato pulp from the insides of your tomatoes. Sprinkle your tomatoes with some salt and allow to stand for at least 30 minutes.

4. Prepare your quinoa according to the directions on the package and once your quinoa is fully cooked, add it to your corn mixture. Toss the ingredients together to combine.

5. Preheat your oven to 350 degrees. While it heats up scoop about ¾ cup of your corn mixture into each of your tomatoes. Sprinkle your cheese on top of each tomato and place into your oven to bake.

6. Bake your tomatoes for 15 minutes. After 15 minutes remove from your oven and set your oven to broil. Broil your tomatoes for an additional 12 minutes or until the cheese fully melts on top. Remove from oven and serve as soon as possible.

4) Early Morning Banana and Berry Parfait

This simple and refreshing breakfast includes protein, grains, and fresh fruit. All ingredients are easy to digest and it involves no cooking.

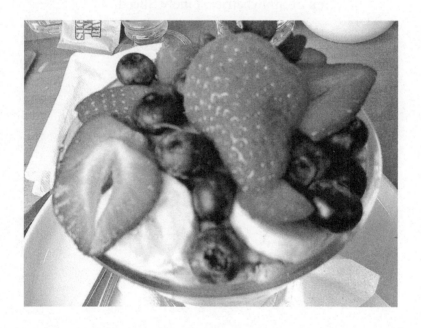

Cooking Time: 1 Hour and 5 Minutes

Makes: 3 to 4 Servings

List of Ingredients:

- ¾ Cup of Blueberries, Fresh
- 1/3 Cup of Granola, Your Favorite Brand
- ½ Of a Banana, Sliced into Small Pieces
- 1 tablespoon of Wheat Germ
- 6 Ounces of Yogurt, Vanilla
- ¾ Cup of Strawberries, Finely Sliced

ssssssssssssssssssssssssssssssssssssssssssssssssss

Procedure:

1. Evenly layer all of your ingredients together into a bowl. Chill for an hour and enjoy.

5) Freshly Buttered Scallops

This is another great recipe to try during your bulletproof protein fasting phase. This is an easy recipe to put together and is a great one to make if you are looking to impress a few people at a dinner party.

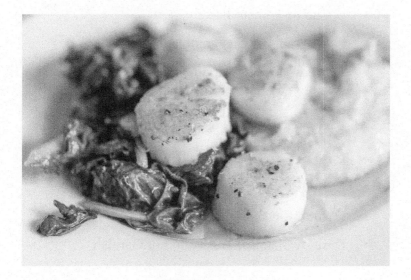

Cooking Time: 15 Minutes

Makes: 3 to 4

List of Ingredients:

- 2 teaspoons of Ginger, Paste and Fresh
- 2 Tablespoons of Coconut Oil
- 2 teaspoons of Garlic, Paste and Fresh
- ½ Cup of Shallots, Fresh and Minced
- ¼ teaspoons of Cumin, Ground
- ¼ Cup of Tomato Paste
- ¼ teaspoons of Cinnamon, Ground
- 1 ½ teaspoons of Garam Masala
- 8 Ounces of Coconut Cream
- 1 Pound of Scallops, Sea, Fresh and Cleaned
- Dash of Sea Salt, For Taste
- Dash of Pepper for Taste
- Dash of Cayenne Pepper for Taste
- Dash of Cilantro, Fresh and For Garnish

SSSSSSSSSSSSSSSSSSSSSSSSSSSSSSSSSSSSSSSSSSSSSSSSS

Procedure:

1. Take out a large wok and heat up your coconut oil over medium to high heat.

2. Then add in your shallots and allow to cook for about 2 to 3 minutes or until the shallots begin to soften.

3. Next add in your tomato paste, ginger paste, garlic paste, garam masala, cumin, cayenne, cinnamon and season with salt and pepper. Stir thoroughly to combine all of the ingredients together. All to cook for an additional 3 to 5 minutes, constantly stirring the entire time.

4. Add in your fresh scallops and your coconut cream to the pan and stir to combine everything. Cook for another 5 minutes or until the scallops are fully cooked through.

5. Remove from heat and sprinkle your fresh cilantro on top of it all. Serve while still piping hot.

6) Tasty Butter and Nut Toast

It doesn't get much easier than the following recipe for toast with Nut butter and toppings. This breakfast is protein dense and extremely quick to prepare.

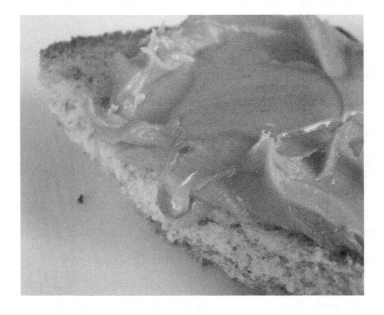

Cooking Time: 5 Minutes

Makes: 1 Serving

List of Ingredients:

- 1 tablespoon of Peanut Butter or Nut Butter, Natural
- 1 Slice of Bread, Your Favorite Brand
- 1 tablespoon of Nuts (Pistachios, Almonds, Peanuts or Cashews), Finely Chopped
- 1 tablespoon of Dried Fruit (Apple, Cherries, Banana, Cranberries), Finely Chopped

sssssssssssssssssssssssssssssssssssssssssssssssssss

Procedure:

1. Top your toasted bread with your natural nut butter.

2. Then top with a sprinkle of nuts and dried fruit. Serve and enjoy.

7) Healthy Pistachio, Apricot and Quinoa Salad

There is nothing healthier than enjoying a quinoa salad for either lunch or dinner. With this dish you will be able to just that while enjoying a dish that will help get you through your busy day

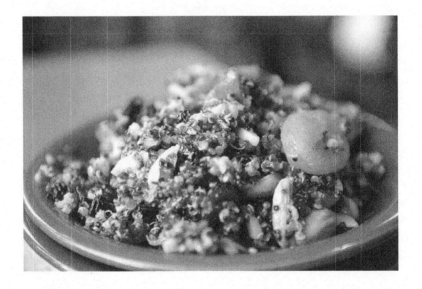

Cooking Time: 30 Minutes

Makes: 4

Ingredients for the Salad:

- 3 Cups of Water
- 1 Cup of Quinoa, Uncooked
- ½ teaspoons of Salt
- 4 Cups of Romaine Lettuce, Thinly Sliced
- 1/3 Cup of Apricots, Dried and Cut into Quarters
- 1/3 Cup of Raisins, Golden in Color
- ¼ Cup of Pistachios, Dry Roasted and Shelled
- ¼ Cup of Green Onions, Finely Sliced
- ¼ Cup of Parsley, Fresh and Chopped Finely
- ¼ Cup of Cilantro, Fresh and Finely Chopped
- 2 Tablespoons of Mint, Fresh and Finely Chopped
- ¼ teaspoons of Black Pepper, Ground

Ingredients for Dressing:

- ½ teaspoons of Lime Rind, Finely Grated
- 2 Tablespoons of Lime Juice, Fresh
- 2 Tablespoons of White Wine, Sweet
- 1 tablespoon of Olive Oil
- ½ to 1 teaspoon of Jalapeno Pepper, Minced
- ¼ teaspoons of Salt
- ¼ teaspoons of Cumin, Ground
- ¼ teaspoons of Coriander, Ground
- ¼ teaspoons of Paprika

ssssssssssssssssssssssssssssssssssssssssssssssssss

Procedure:

1. To make your salad you will first want to cook your quinoa. To do this place your quinoa into a medium sized saucepan with some water and allow to come to a boil. Once it is boiling, reduce the heat to a low simmer and allow the quinoa to cook for an additional 15 minutes.

2. Then remove your mixture from heat and fluff with a fork. Then combine your cooked quinoa with all of your ingredients for your salad and toss lightly to combine all of the ingredients. Set aside.

3. To prepare your dressing for your salad combine all of your ingredients together in a small sized mixing bowl and whisk with a whisk until it is a smooth consistency.

4. To serve, add a generous amount of your quinoa salad to a salad plate and top with some dressing. Serve immediately and enjoy.

8) Classic Zucchini Fritte

The zucchini is crisp and light in texture and taste. They may be served with your favorite tomato sauce for dipping.

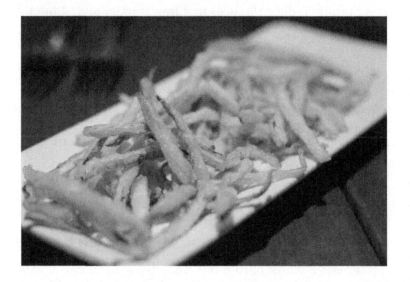

Cooking Time: 20 Minutes

Makes: 4 to 6

List of Ingredients:

- 3 Zucchini, Fresh and Cut into Thin Slices
- 1 Cup of Bread Crumbs
- ¼ Cup of Parmesan Cheese, Finely Grated
- 2 teaspoons Of Garlic Powder
- ½ teaspoons of Black Pepper
- 1 teaspoon of Parsley, Dried
- ½ teaspoons of Oregano, Dried
- 2 Eggs, Large in Size and Beaten
- 1 Cup of Olive oil
- Dash of Salt
- Dash of Paprika

sssssssssssssssssssssssssssssssssssssssssssssssss

Procedure:

For Prep:

1. Mix together your breadcrumbs, Parmesan, garlic powder, pepper, parsley, and oregano, and in a medium sized mixing bowl until thoroughly mixed then place into a shallow dish.

2. Next dip your fresh zucchini slices into your beaten eggs then into your bread crumbs. Make sure that you press them gently and roll them to make sure that you cover all of the sides.

3. Then place your zucchini slices onto a clean plate in one single layer.

For Cooking:

1. Heat up your olive oil in a large sized skillet over medium to high heat. Once the oil is very hot, fry up each zucchini slice until it is golden in color and crisp. This should take about 3 to 4 minutes. As they cook make sure that you turn the slice halfway through cooking.

2. Drain your fully cooked zucchini slices on paper towels and sprinkle with a dash of paprika, and serve with a side of fresh tomato sauce for dipping. Enjoy.

9) Traditional BBQ Pulled Pork

Slowly roasting the pork keeps the meat tender and it shreds easily. Placing it in the smoker adds another layer of flavor. The All-Purpose Cider BBQ Sauce complements the pork nicely.

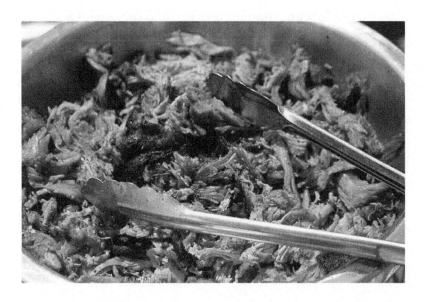

Cooking Time: 5 to 7 Hours and 30 Minutes

Makes: 5 to 7 Pounds of Pulled Pork

List of Ingredients:

- 3 Tablespoons of Paprika
- 2 Tablespoons of Garlic Powder
- 2 Tablespoons of Brown Sugar, Packed
- 5 to 7 Pounds of Pork, Shoulder or Butt
- 2 Tablespoons of Mustard Powder
- 2 Tablespoons of Salt for Taste
- Some Hamburger Buns
- 3 to 4 Cups of Wood Chips, Mesquite Preferable

sssssssssssssssssssssssssssssssssssssssssssssssssss

Procedure:

1. Mix your dry ingredients together until they are evenly blended. Then rinse and dry your pork and rub your spice blend all over the pork. Marinate your pork for at least 1 hour or overnight in your refrigerator.

2. Prepare your smoker according to the manufacturer's instructions and your wood chips. Your smoker temperature should be at least 225 degrees. Place your pork into your smoker and cook for about 5 to 7 hours or until the internal temperature reaches 160 degrees.

3. Allow your pork to rest for a couple of minutes then place your pork on a large cutting board. Use two forks to pull the meat apart in shreds from your roast.

To serve, place your pork on a toasted bun and pour on your favorite BBQ sauce and enjoy.

10) Fresh and Healthy Ginger Muffins

These ginger muffins make an easy snack that you can enjoy on the run. Ginger is one of the best and most natural ingredients to use to combat morning sickness. So if you are having a queasy stomach, this is the perfect snack to have to make you feel better.

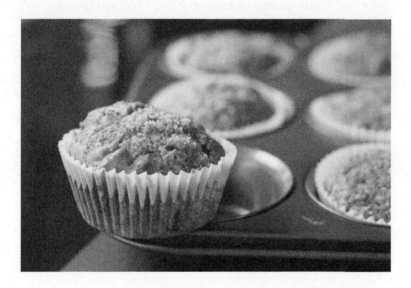

Cooking Time: 30 Minutes

Makes: 16 Muffins

List of Ingredients:

- 2 Cups of Flour, All Purpose
- ½ teaspoons of Salt, For Taste
- ¾ Cup Plus 3 Tablespoons of Sugar, White
- ½ Cup of Butter
- ¾ teaspoons of Baking Soda
- 2 Eggs, Large in Size
- 1 Cup of Buttermilk
- 2 Tablespoons of Lemon Zest, Freshly Grated
- 2 Ounces of Ginger Root, Unpeeled

SSSSSSSSSSSSSSSSSSSSSSSSSSSSSSSSSSSSSSSSSSSSSSSSSSSSS

Procedure:

1. Preheat your oven to 375 degrees. While your oven is preheating grease up 2 medium sized muffin pans.

2. Then chop up your ginger into very fine pieces.

3. Next place your ¾ cup of sugar into a medium sized saucepan over medium heat and stir until the sugar fully dissolves. Set aside and allow to cool for a couple of minutes.

4. Then using a food processor, combine your freshly grated lemon zest and remaining tablespoon of sugar. Then add your sugar and lemon zest mixture to your ginger mixture and stir thoroughly combined.

5. Beat your butter next and ½ cup sugar in a medium sized mixing bowl until smooth in consistency. Then add in your eggs and continue beating until thoroughly combined. While continuing to mix, slowly add the following ingredients in this order: buttermilk, flour, salt, and baking soda.

6. Add in your lemon-ginger mixture and stir thoroughly by hand until combined.

7. Fill each muffin cup approximately ¾ full with the mixture.

8. Place into your preheated oven to bake for at least 15-20 minutes. Remove from oven and serve warm or store for easy to grab breakfasts. Enjoy.

11) Italian Style Egg Drop Soup

Pouring the beaten eggs into the hot broth creates delicate strings of cooked egg. It is seasoned with a few simple and fresh flavors.

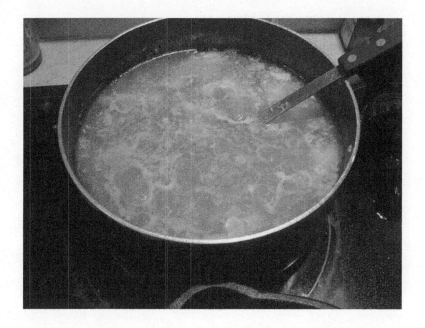

Cooking Time: 15 Minutes

Makes: 2

List of Ingredients:

- 5 Cups of Chicken Stock
- 2 Large Sized Eggs, Beaten Lightly
- 4 Tablespoons of Parmesan, Finely Shaved
- ¼ Cup of Fresh Italian Parsley, Finely Chopped
- 1 teaspoon Of Marjoram
- 1 tablespoon of Lemon Zest, Fresh
- Dash of Sea Salt
- Dash of Parmesan, Fine Shavings

sssssssssssssssssssssssssssssssssssssssssssssssssssss

Procedure:

1. Bring your chicken stock to a rolling boil in a large sized saucepan. Then reduce the heat to low and slowly add in your beaten eggs by drizzling them into your chicken stock.

2. Next add in your parsley, marjoram, and fresh lemon zest. Of course you will want to adjust your seasoning with a dash of salt and pepper for taste. Serve immediately and garnish with fresh Parmesan shavings. Enjoy!

12) Crockpot Style Oatmeal

What could be easier than waking up to breakfast already made? Oatmeal is a natural immune system booster and contains fiber and antioxidants.

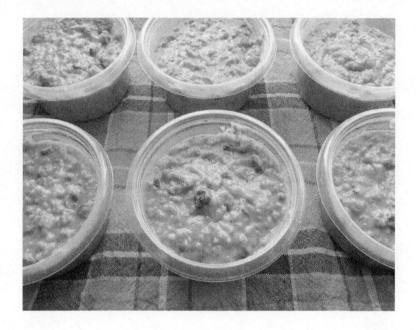

Cooking Time: 6 to 8 Hours

Makes: 4

List of Ingredients:

- 3 Cups of Water, Warm
- 1 Cup of Oats, Fresh
- 1 Pinch of Salt, For Taste
- 1 Cup of Half and Half
- ¼ Cup of Brown Sugar

sssssssssssssssssssssssssssssssssssssssssssssssssssss

Procedure:

1. Mix together your oats and water in your crock pot until combined thoroughly.

2. Then set on the lowest setting and allow to cook covered throughout the night, while you sleep.

3. In the morning, add in your remaining ingredients and stir. Enjoy.

13) Arugula and Potato Omelet

With a few sautéed potatoes and an abundance of chopped arugula, this dish combines a perfect combination or nutty and peppery omelets. Since the arugula is cooked only a few seconds, it retains its bright green hue and adds a bit of texture. Have all the ingredients for the filling ready before you start to make the omelets, and then count on less than 5 minutes from start to finish for each one.

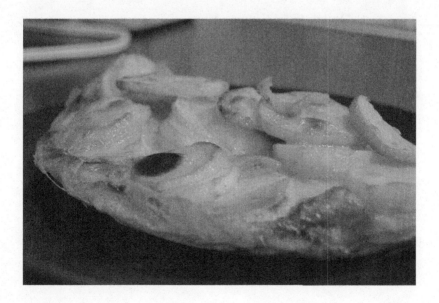

Cooking Time: 15 Minutes

Makes: 2

List of Ingredients:

- ½ Tablespoons of Olive Oil
- 2 ½ Tablespoons of Butter, Unsalted
- Dash of Salt and Black Pepper for Taste
- 4 Eggs, Large in Size
- 1 teaspoon of Cayenne Pepper
- 4 Ounce of Potatoes, Res, Scrubbed and Sliced in Small Cubes
- 8 Cups of Arugula, Fresh, Stems Chopped, Washed, Drained and Chopped
- ½ Tablespoons of Vinegar, Balsamic
- 6 Tablespoons of Gruyere Cheese, Grated

sssssssssssssssssssssssssssssssssssssssssssssssssss

Procedure:

1. Heat up your ½ Tablespoons of butter in a medium sized saucepan with some olive oil. Set over medium heat. Once the pan is hot add in your potatoes and sauté for the next 8 minutes or until light golden brown in color. Remove from heat and season with a dash of salt and pepper. Set aside.

2. Then whisk your eggs in a medium sized mixing bowl. Season with a dash of salt and cayenne pepper.

3. Then using another medium sized mixing bowl, add in your arugula and toss with some vinegar. Using separate bowls place your Gruyere cheese and potatoes into them.

4. Next add in 1 tablespoon of Butter into a medium sized frying pan and set over medium heat. When the pan is hot ladle in half of your egg mix into it and stir until the eggs begin to set but are still liquid in state. Using a spatula lift up the edges of your omelet and allow the uncooked portion to run underneath to cook. You will want to repeat this for about 2 or 3 more times until the eggs are fully cooked.

5. Next sprinkle in half of your potato mixture, cheese and arugula over your eggs. Allow the mix to cook until the cheese begins to melt and the arugula begins to wilt slightly. This should take about 30 seconds.

6. Then fold your omelet in half and slide it gently onto a serving plate. Repeat to make your second omelet. Serve and enjoy the moment it touches the plate.

14) Delicious Egg Soufflé with Spinach, Ricotta and Pancetta

This dish is relatively simple to prepare, and it is absolutely delectable. With its striking presentation this dish uses a custard base of eggs, cream, and ricotta is combined with chopped spinach and sautéed pancetta and then poured over toasted bread cubes to make a mouthwatering dish that you will fall in love with.

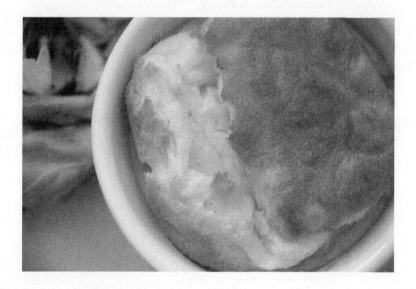

Cooking Time: 50 Minutes

Makes: 5 to 6

List of Ingredients:

- Some Unsalted Butter, For Greasing
- 2 Ounces of Baguette Slices, With the Crusts Removed
- 8 Eggs, Large in Size
- 1 Cup of Heavy Cream
- ¼ teaspoons of Salt, Kosher
- 1 ½ Tablespoons of Olive Oil
- ½ Cup of Ricotta, Whole Milk
- ½ teaspoons of Nutmeg, Freshly Grated
- 2 Pinches of Black Pepper for Taste
- 1 Pinch of Cayenne Pepper
- 1 ½ Cups of Baby Spinach, Chopped Roughly
- 4 Ounces of Pancetta, Sliced into Cubes and Fried Until Crispy

sssssssssssssssssssssssssssssssssssssssssssssssss

Procedure:

1. Preheat your oven to 375 degrees. Make sure that you arrange your racks so that one sits right in the center of your oven. While your oven heats up grease up a medium sized baking dish with some of your butter.

2. Then place your sliced bread cubes into a medium sized bowl. Toss with a touch of olive oil to coat your bread evenly. Then spread your cubes of bread onto a medium sized baking sheet and place into your oven. Bake for the next 5 minutes until golden brown in color. Remove from oven and spread into your baking dish.

3. Next using a large sized mixing bowl whisk your eggs until they are completely beaten. Then whisk together your cream, pepper, nutmeg, salt, ricotta and cayenne pepper until thoroughly blended. Then add in your spinach and pancetta until thoroughly mixed.

4. Place your dish into your oven and bake the mixture for about 30 to 40 minutes. Remove from your oven and allow to cool for the next 5 minutes before serving and enjoying.

15) Delicious Grilled Balsamic Vegetable Salad

If you are looking for a salad recipe that will enhance the natural flavor and sweetness of your veggies, this is the salad recipe for you. While still preserving all of the important nutrients this recipe will bring you a dish that tastes smoky and is absolutely delicious.

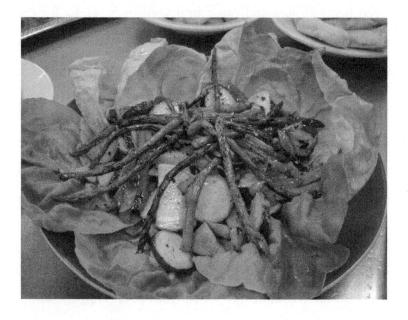

Cooking Time: 35 Minutes

Makes: 6 Servings

List of Ingredients:

- 1 Zucchini, Fresh and Sliced Thinly
- 1 Eggplant, Fresh, Peeled and Sliced Thinly
- 2 Tomatoes, Ripe and Sliced Finely
- 1 Carrot, Fresh and Cut Lengthwise Very Finely
- 1 Onion, Red in Color and Sliced Finely
- 2 Yellow Bell Pepper, Fresh, Cored and Sliced into Quarters
- 2 Tablespoons of Olive Oil
- ¼ Cup of Vinegar, Balsamic
- Dash of Salt and Pepper for Taste
- 4 Cloves of Garlic, Chopped Finely

sssssssssssssssssssssssssssssssssssssssssssssssssss

Procedure:

1. Using a medium sized saucepan, heat it over high heat and place all of your vegetables into it, one by one.

2. Sauté your veggies until they are brown on each side and then remove from heat. Place them into a medium sized mixing bowl.

3. Using a separate bowl mix up your balsamic vinegar, dash of salt and pepper for taste, olive oil and garlic together until evenly combined.

4. Pour your new dressing over your grilled veggies and serve immediately. Enjoy.

16) Tasty Eggplant Parmesan

Eggplant Parmesan is one of the most popular and favorite Italian appetizers that there is. The texture is both crispy and chewy, making this an appetizer that everyone will fall in love within your home.

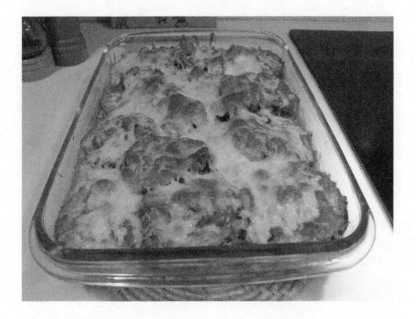

Cooking Time: 40 Minutes

Makes: 4

List of Ingredients:

- 1 Eggplant, Large in Size, Peeled and Sliced Thinly
- ⅓ Cup of Milk
- ⅓ Cup of Italian Breadcrumbs
- ½ Cup of Olive Oil
- 1 ½ Cup of Tomato Sauce, Fresh
- ⅓ Cup of Parmesan Cheese, Finely Grated Plus Extra for Topping
- Some Basil leaves

sssssssssssssssssssssssssssssssssssssssssssssssssssss

Procedure:

For Preparation:

1. First preheat your oven to 400 degrees. While your oven heats up salt your eggplant slices on both sides generously. Allow them to rest for about 15 to 20 minutes. This will help to get rid of any excess moisture that may be trapped in the eggplant.

2. Then place your eggplant into a strainer. Using a few paper towels carefully wipe the salt and water off your eggplant slices, making sure that you wipe both sides.

3. Next dip your sliced eggplant into your milk, then coat with your breadcrumbs, making sure to cover both sides. Then place them in a single layer on a separate dish until all of the slices have been thorough coated.

4. Then heat up some olive oil in a large sized skillet over medium to high heat. Once the oil is very hot, reduce your heat to medium and cook each eggplant slice for about 2 minutes on each side or until it turns golden brown in color.

For Cooking:

1. Using a medium sized baking dish, spoon some tomato sauce onto each eggplant slice, and top each slice with a generous amount of Parmesan cheese.

2. Place into your oven to bake for about 10 to 12 minutes or until it becomes bubbly.

3. Remove from oven. To serve your slices make sure that you garnish each slice with some fresh basil leaves, and sprinkle with a generous amount Parmesan cheese. Serve and enjoy.

17) Perfect Lunchtime Spinach and Avocado Salad

The best part about this salad can be either the rich flavor of the poppy seeds that you use for the dressing or the creamy texture of the avocado. The contrast between these two ingredients help make this a dish that is both filling and delicious.

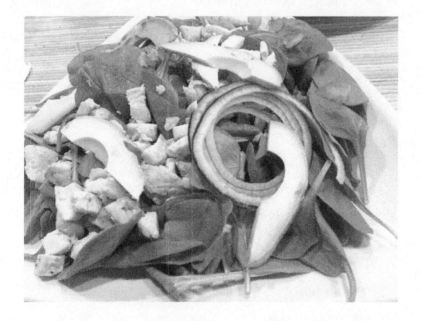

Cooking Time: 20 Minutes

Makes: 6 Servings

List of Ingredients:

- 2 Tablespoons of Almonds, Sliced
- 1 Pound of Spinach, Baby
- 1 Avocado, Ripe, peeled and sliced
- 1 tablespoon of Poppy Seeds
- ½ of A Lemon, juiced
- 1 teaspoon of Honey
- 1 teaspoon of Lemon Zest, Fresh
- 1 tablespoon of Olive Oil
- Dash of Salt and Pepper for Taste
- 1 teaspoon of Vinegar, Apple Cider

sssssssssssssssssssssssssssssssssssssssssssssssss

Procedure:

1. In a salad bowl combine your avocado, spinach and almonds until gently mixed together.

2. In a small sized mixing bowl combine the rest of your ingredients together to make your dressing. Stir together until thoroughly mixed.

3. Drizzle your dressing over your salad and serve while as fresh as possible.

18) Surprisingly Healthy Zucchini Muffins

Adding vegetables to muffins is an easy way to get some added nutrition at a time when morning sickness is making it difficult to eat.

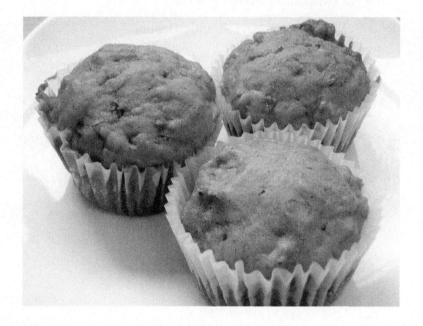

Cooking Time: 35 to 40 Minutes

Makes: 12 Muffins

List of Ingredients:

- 3 Cups of Flour, All Purpose
- ½ teaspoons of Nutmeg, Ground
- 2 teaspoons of Cinnamon, Ground
- ½ teaspoons of Salt
- ¼ Cup of Brown Sugar, Light and Packed
- 2 teaspoons of Baking Soda
- 2 Eggs, Large and Slightly Beaten
- 3 Cups of Zucchini, Fresh and Grated
- 1 Cup of Raisins
- 2 teaspoons of Vanilla
- 2/3 Cup of Canola Oil
- 1 Cup of Pecans, Finely Chopped

sssssssssssssssssssssssssssssssssssssssssssssssssssss

Procedure:

1. Preheat your oven to 350 degrees.

2. Next whisk together your brown sugar, vanilla, and eggs in a medium sized mixing bowl. Then mix your zucchini, oil, salt, and baking soda.

3. Then combine your flour with your nutmeg and cinnamon in a separate small sized bowl. Next you will then want to mix your two bowls of ingredients together until thoroughly combined. Then add in your pecans and raisins.

4. Fill your greased up muffin tins about ¾ of the way with your batter.

5. Place your muffins into your preheated oven to bake for the next 25-30 minutes. Remove from oven and serve when you are ready.

19) Classic Thai Style Tomato Soup

While this tomato soup looks anything but different when you first look at it, but the moment that you taste it for the first time you will immediately taste all of those wonderful Thai flavors that will send your taste buds straight to heaven. There is no need to add anything more to this dish as it already has everything you are looking for.

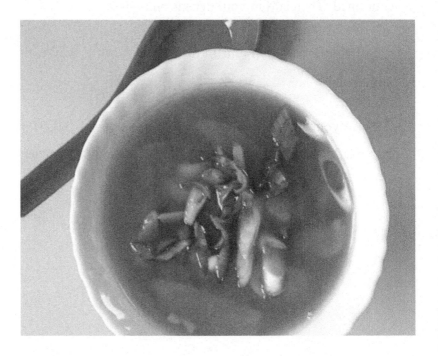

Cooking Time: 45 Minutes

Makes: 6 Servings

List of Ingredients:

- 2 Tablespoons of Olive Oil
- 1 Shallot, Medium in Size and Chopped Finely
- 2 Cloves of Garlic, Finely Chopped
- 12 Inches of Grass Stalk, Lemon and Crushed
- 4 Tomatoes, Heirloom, Peeled and Chopped Finely
- 1 teaspoon of Ginger, Grated
- Dash of Salt and Pepper
- 3 Cups of Vegetable Stock
- 1 teaspoon of Hot Sauce, Your Favorite Brand

sssssssssssssssssssssssssssssssssssssssssssssssssssss

Procedure:

1. Using a large sized soup pot, heat up your olive oil over medium to high heat and then add in your minced garlic and chopped shallot. Sauté these for the next 2 minutes or until fragrant.

2. Then add in the rest of your ingredients and allow the soup to cook for the next 20 to 25 minutes.

3. Remove from heat and toss out your lemongrass stalk. Pour your soup into a blender and puree your soup until it reaches the desired consistency that you want.

4. Pour your soup into serving bowls and serve either warm or chilled. Enjoy.

20) Sweet Citrus Salad and Ginger Yogurt

This simple breakfast, which can be made ahead of time, is refreshing and contains high amounts of vitamin C. The ginger in the recipe is great for women who are especially suffering from morning sickness within the first trimester or their pregnancy.

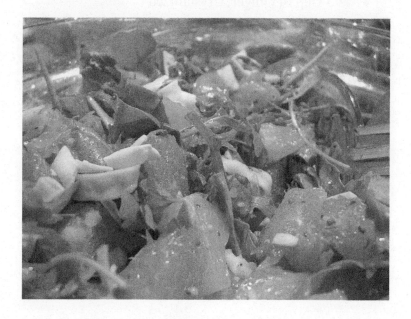

Cooking Time: 10 Minutes

Makes: 6 Servings

List of Ingredients:

- ½ Cup of Cranberries, Dried
- 16 Ounces of Yogurt, Greek
- 1 Grapefruit, Fresh, Peeled and Chopped into Tiny Pieces
- 2 Tangerines, Large in Size, Peeled and Chopped into Tiny Pieces
- 2 Tablespoons of Honey, Raw
- 2/3 Cup of Ginger, Crystallized
- ¼ teaspoons of Cinnamon, Ground
- 3 Oranges, Naval, Peeled and Chopped into Tiny Pieces

ssssssssssssssssssssssssssssssssssssssssssssssssss

Procedure:

1. Place your chopped citrus fruit into a small serving bowl and mix in your dried cranberries or use raisins if you wish.

2. Add in your honey and ground cinnamon next. Place into your refrigerator for at least 1 hour.

3. While you wait for your refrigerated mixture waiting, combine your yogurt and ginger together in a separate small sized bowl.

4. Once you are ready to eat, spoon your yogurt mixture on top of your citrus fruit mixture and enjoy.

21) Eggs, Leeks and Bacon Alla Gratin

Feel free to assemble this dish the night before you decide to prepare it if it makes it easier for you. This dish incorporates toasted French bread, sautéed leeks, crispy fried bacon, and bits of creamy St. André are all combined with a savory mixture of eggs and half-and-half, making it a dish that will soon become a fan favorite in your household

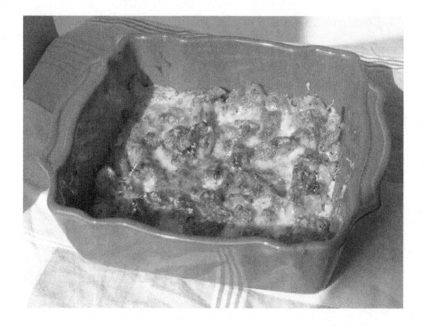

Cooking Time: 55 Minutes

Makes: 6

List of Ingredients:

- Some Unsalted Butter, For Greasing
- 1 Whole Baguette, Your Favorite Kind
- 2 Cups of Leeks, Chopped Finely
- 6 Eggs, Large in Size
- 6 Slices of Bacon, Thick Cut
- 2 ½ Cups of Half and Half
- 6 Ounces of St. Andre Cheese, Chilled
- ½ teaspoons of Salt
- 2 Pinches of Cayenne Pepper
- 1 tablespoon of Parsley, Minced

sssssssssssssssssssssssssssssssssssssssssssssssssss

Procedure:

1. Preheat your oven to 350 degrees. While the oven heats up arrange your racks so that you have one in the very center of your oven and grease a medium sized baking dish with your butter.

2. Cut your baguette into small slices and place in your baking dish to form a single layer. You should use about 20 to 25 slices. If you have any leftover set aside to use at another time. Place your slices into your oven and allow to bake for about 10 minutes, making sure to flip the bread halfway through.

3. While those bakes take out a medium sized frying pan and set it over medium heat. Fry up your bacon until they are crisp and browned. This should take about 5 minutes. Once done drain on a paper towel and set aside.

4. Using the same frying pan with a touch of the bacon grease left over, add in your leeks and cook them until they begin to soften. This should take about 4 minutes. Remove from heat.

5. Then sprinkle your cooked bacon and leeks over your bread slices in your baking dish.

6. Next cut your cheese into small cubes and scatter them over your bread in the bacon dish.

7. Then using a medium sized mixing bowl whisk your eggs with your half and half, cayenne pepper and salt. Pour this mixture into your baking dish. Cover with some plastic wrap and allow to sit for 1 hour or 24 hours for the best results.

8. After 24 hours bake your dish until the eggs are fully set and the top is golden brown in color. This will take about 40 to 45 minutes. Remove from oven and allow to cool for 5 minutes.

8. Season with your minced parsley and serve while it is still piping hot. Enjoy.

22) Mouthwatering Bacon Stuffed Cheeseburgers

Texans are particular about the proper burger patty. Simply, grilled burgers taste best with ground chuck. Many try to use sirloin or round, but 80/ 20 chuck gives you maximum flavor and moistness in the grilled hamburger. This recipe has some of the "fixin's" on the inside. Pile your favorite toppings on after they come off the grill.

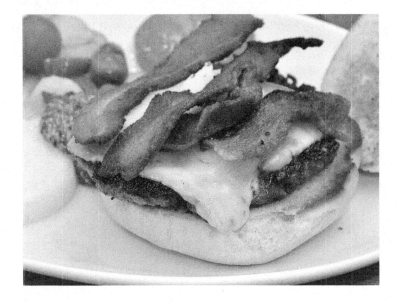

Cooking Time: 20 Minutes

Makes: 4 Large Cheeseburgers

List of Ingredients:

- 2 Pounds of Ground Chuck, 80/20 Preferable
- 2 Ounces of Cheddar Cheese, White and Sliced Into 4 Slices
- 2 Ounces of Pepper Jack Cheese, Sliced Into 4 Slices
- 8 Strips of Bacon, Fully Cooked Until Crisp
- Dash of Black Pepper for Taste
- Dash of Garlic Powder for Taste
- Touch of Vegetable Oil
- 4 Hamburger Buns
- Condiments and Toppings of Your Choice
- Some Wax Paper

sssssssssssssssssssssssssssssssssssssssssssssssss

Procedure:

1. Divide your chuck into 8 even pieces. The secret is to form 8 very thin patties. Place your chuck portions onto your wax paper and cover with some additional wax paper. Then using the bottom of a heavy skillet as a press, press your chuck to about 1/ 4" thinness. Sprinkle each of your patties with some black pepper and garlic powder for taste.

2. Assemble 2 strips of your crumbled bacon and 1 piece of each type cheese in the very center of your patties. Be sure that your ingredients do not hang over the edges of the patties. Then place your other 4 patties on top. Re-cover with your wax paper and gently press around the edges to make a tight seal. Brush your patties with some vegetable oil on both sides.

3. Next, cook your patties on a hot grill. Do not flip your patties more than once. Cook for about 5 to 7 minutes on each side of your patty for medium to well done. Serve immediately and enjoy.

23) Mini Spinach Pizza

It is no secret that spinach is one of the healthiest vegetables that you can have today. However, it is hard to include in everyone's diet simply because to many people it does not taste good. With this recipe you do not have to worry about that because who doesn't love a great tasting pizza?

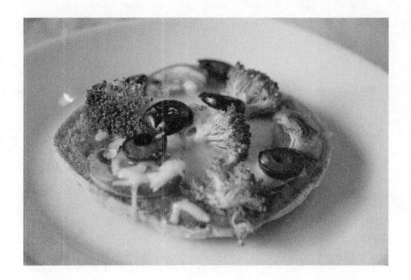

Cooking Time: 30 Minutes

Makes: 6 Servings

List of Ingredients:

- 6 Pita Breads, Whole Wheat
- ½ Cup of Tomato Sauce, Fresh or Canned
- 1 Cup of Spinach Leaves, Fresh and Left Whole
- 1 Cup of Mozzarella Cheese, Fresh and Shredded
- Dash of Salt and Pepper for Taste

ssssssssssssssssssssssssssssssssssssssssssssssssssss

Procedure:

1. Preheat your oven to 350 degrees. While your oven heats up place your whole grain pita bread onto a baking sheet.

2. Brush each pita bread slice with your fresh tomato sauce and cover with a layer of fresh spinach and shredded mozzarella cheese. Season with your dash of salt and pepper.

3. Place your baking sheet into your oven and allow to bake for the next 10 to 15 minutes or until the mozzarella has fully melted and the tops are crusty.

4. Remove from oven and either serve immediately or serve once completely chilled. Enjoy.

24) Tasty Cucumber and Cream Cheese Cups

This is a great idea for a recipe especially if you are looking to serve a fresh appetizer that is incredibly low in calories. The filling that you will use in this recipe is low in fat and tastes great, allowing you and your baby to enjoy this dish without having to feel guilty about it.

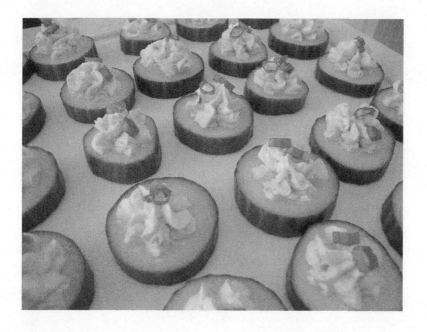

Cooking Time: 30 Minutes

Makes: 4 Servings

List of Ingredients:

- 2 Cucumbers, Fresh and Sliced into Thick Slices
- ½ Cup of Cream Cheese, Low in Fat and Softened
- 1 Clove of Garlic, Minced
- 1 tablespoon of Dill, Finely Chopped
- 1 tablespoon of Parsley, Finely Chopped
- Dash of Salt and Pepper for Taste

sssssssssssssssssssssssssssssssssssssssssssssssssss

Procedure:

1. Slice up your fresh cucumber and scoop out some of the flesh of the cucumber to help form your "cups." Place the "cups" onto a serving dish.

2. In a small sized mixing bowl mix together your parsley, cream cheese, dill and garlic together until evenly mixed. Next add your dash of salt and pepper for taste and spoon the mixture into your "cups."

3. Serve while still fresh and enjoy immediately.

25) Fresh Mozzarella and Tomato on a Stick

This is one of the fastest appetizer recipes that you will ever make. They look beautiful and are packed full of fresh taste, giving you a dish that you won't soon forget. While it may be a simple recipe to make, this is a dish that will certainly shine at your dinner table.

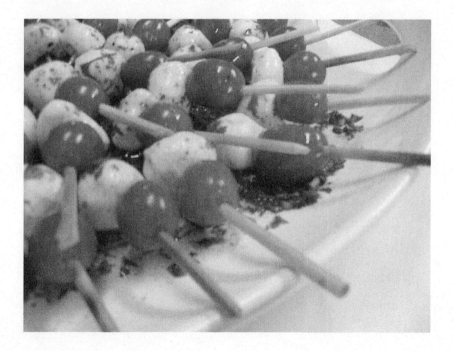

Cooking Time: 20 Minutes

Makes: 6 Servings

List of Ingredients:

- 2 Cups of Tomatoes, Cherry and Fresh
- 6 Ounces of Mozzarella, Fresh and Cut into Small Cubes or Balls
- 6 Leaves of Basil, Fresh
- Dash of Salt and Pepper for Taste
- 2 Tablespoons of Olive Oil
- A Handful of Skewers or Toothpicks, Wooden

sssssssssssssssssssssssssssssssssssssssssssssssss

Procedure:

1. Gently place your fresh mozzarella and tomatoes onto your wooden skewers or toothpicks.

2. Then garnish your skewers with your basil leaves and dash of salt and pepper. Place them onto a serving plate and drizzle with a touch of olive oil. Serve immediately and enjoy.

26) Savory Minestrone Soup

This is an easy soup that is very traditional and very satisfying. Serve with crusty bread for dunking.

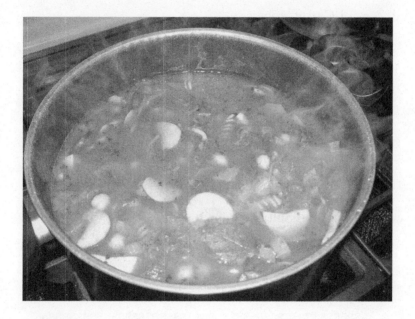

Cooking Time: 20 Minutes

Makes: 3 to 4

List of Ingredients:

- 2 Tablespoons of Olive Oil
- 1 Medium Sized Potato, Diced Finely
- 2 Tablespoons of Onion, Diced Finely
- 1 Carrot, cubed
- 1 Celery Stalk, Sliced
- 2 Cloves of Garlic, Peeled and Sliced
- 1 Cup of Zucchini, Diced
- 2 Cans of Low-Sodium Chicken Broth
- 1 Can of Cannelloni Beans
- 1 Can of Italian-Style Stewed Tomatoes
- Dash of Salt and Pepper
- 1 Cup of Small Pasta, Uncooked
- Some Parmesan cheeses

SSSSSSSSSSSSSSSSSSSSSSSSSSSSSSSSSSSSSSSSSSSSSSSSSSSSSSSS

Procedure:

1. In a medium sized saucepan, heat up your olive oil over medium to high heat then add in your potato, onion, and carrot. Cook your veggies for about 5 to 7 minutes or until your vegetables are soft.

2. Then add all of your remaining ingredients into your saucepan except for your pasta, and bring your mixture to a rolling boil.

3. Then reduce the heat and add in your pasta. Cook until your pasta becomes tender and al dente. Season your freshly made minestrone soup with a dash salt and pepper for taste.

4. Serve evenly into soup bowls and top with a generous amount of Parmesan cheese. Enjoy.

About the Author

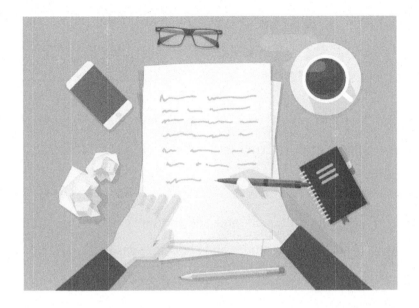

Allie Allen developed her passion for the culinary arts at the tender age of five when she would help her mother cook for their large family of 8. Even back then, her family knew this would be more than a hobby for the young Allie and when she graduated from high school, she applied to cooking school in London. It had always been a dream of the young chef to study with some of Europe's best and she made it happen by attending the Chef Academy of London.

After graduation, Allie decided to bring her skills back to North America and open up her own restaurant. After 10 successful years as head chef and owner, she decided to sell her business and pursue other career avenues. This monumental decision led Allie to her true calling, teaching. She also started to write e-books for her students to study at home for practice. She is now the proud author of several e-books and gives private and semi-private cooking lessons to a range of students at all levels of experience.

Stay tuned for more from this dynamic chef and teacher when she releases more informative e-books on cooking and baking in the near future. Her work is infused with stores and anecdotes you will love!

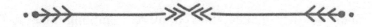

Author's Afterthoughts

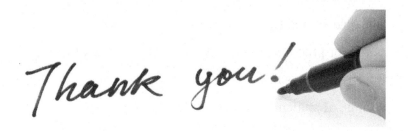

I can't tell you how grateful I am that you decided to read my book. My most heartfelt thanks that you took time out of your life to choose my work and I hope you find benefit within these pages.

There are so many books available today that offer similar content so that makes it even more humbling that you decided to buying mine.

Tell me what you thought! I am eager to hear your opinion and ideas on what you read as are others who are looking for a good book to buy. Leave a review on Amazon.com so others can benefit from your wisdom!

With much thanks,

Allie Allen